THE
EPIPHYSIS

Alan Gilchrist

AuthorHouse™ UK
1663 Liberty Drive
Bloomington, IN 47403 USA
www.authorhouse.co.uk
UK TFN: 0800 0148641 (Toll Free inside the UK)
UK Local: 02036 956322 (+44 20 3695 6322 from outside the UK)

Because of the dynamic nature of the Internet, any web addresses or links contained in this book may have changed since publication and may no longer be valid. The views expressed in this work are solely those of the author and do not necessarily reflect the views of the publisher, and the publisher hereby disclaims any responsibility for them.

Any people depicted in stock imagery provided by Getty Images are models, and such images are being used for illustrative purposes only.
Certain stock imagery © Getty Images.

This book is printed on acid-free paper.

ISBN: 979-8-8230-8976-0 (sc)
ISBN: 979-8-8230-8977-7 (e)

Library of Congress Control Number: 2024919265

Print information available on the last page.

Published by AuthorHouse 09/16/2024

authorHOUSE

Dedication

To my son Andrew and his wife Kim, who live in Oswestry, I thank them for many years of comfort they gave me after returning to England in 2013. To Graham Jones, a sheep farmer near Oswestry, who gave me several stillborn lambs, I am grateful. These were of vital importance to the confirmation of the similarity between the circulation in the human foetus, and that of the sheep foetus, both of which I had discovered in Africa .I am also grateful to Kevin Battams of Battams butchery Oswestry, for providing me with parts of a lamb,s anatomy, as I had asked. These allowed me to see the difference between the lamb's anatomy and that of the foetus, and to suggest what may happen at birth. I thank my friend John Quinn, a professional photographer, who came out of retirement and helped me with my book in many ways. Another friend who deserves my thanks is Ben Hillidge, an IT specialist whose contribution complimented John's. After my stroke in June 2022, my daughter Mary Kirkman, invited me to stay with her husband Bernard and family in Horley, It was a happy move. Mary has helped a lot with the secretarial work. After several years of divorce from AuthorHouse UK, we are now happily reunited, with the outcome you may see in the following pages. I must not forget to thank the DWP for the generous financial support it has given me ever since I returned from Africa in 2013.

Between 1963 and 1967 I was the Medical Superintendent in the hospital of the small Rhodesian town of Fort Victoria. The normal complement of doctors was two, but for three of the four years I worked there I was single-handed. Then in addition to the widest range of my clinical work, which often included major surgery, I became involved in a huge amount of forensic medical work for the Police, and the combination of the two was to develop into a unique medical experience without equal: four years of forensic medicine side by side with four years of clinical medicine of great diversity. The patients came from a large part of the Victoria Province and all the forensic cases which occurred in the province were managed by the police in Fort Victoria. There were three forensic categories: night calls to examine drunken drivers, victims of assault and rape; the collection of human remains from the countryside, and police post-mortems. The night calls were frequent, the post-mortems numerous, and the trips to the countryside happened four times. On each occasion I was escorted by the police after I had finished the hospital work. The last trip was to a grave, many miles away. A teen-aged girl had died under suspicious circumstances three months previously and the police had been informed. The magistrate then issued me with an order to exhume the body. When we started out it was daylight, but we arrived in the dark. The digging was carried out by the police under the headlights of the police vehicle, reflected down from a spare aluminium petrol can from the police vehicle, and held by me. When parts of the skeleton, wrapped in a cloth, became visible I jumped into the grave and helped the others to remove them.

I was unable to find a cause for the death of the girl from my examination of the skeleton, and after the court case the relatives allowed me to keep the skeleton. The date of the exhumation would have been about 1965, and the skeleton has been in my possession for more than 50 years. In May 1967 I was posted from Fort Victoria to Salisbury, the Capital, now known as Harare. At the end of 1969 I resigned from the Rhodesian medical service and on 1st April 1970 opened my own general medical practice in the suburb of Greendale, about ten miles away from the city centre. In December 1967, when I was still in the medical service, I began to draw the vertebrae of the skeleton in Indian ink. On 6th February 1968 I had drawn two views of the 9th dorsal vertebra and stopped the drawing. I completed it 16 years later, on 21st March 1984, when I was in private practice, and finished the drawings of all the vertebrae on 12th September 1984. Before leaving Zimbabwe at the end of June 2013, I visited the officials in the Ministry of Health to obtain a certificate to export the skeleton. They said they would contact me, but they did not do so. I wrapped up the bones separately in strips of cloth and let them go by sea with the rest of my heavy luggage. I was so interested in the skeleton and wanted to bring it over to England because it was a rare and valuable one: the epiphyses were present on many of the bones. I knew I would not be satisfied until I had understood why we have epiphyses.

I have had an unusually wide range of experience with the use of a microscope. Each student had to have a microscope for the biology classes in medical school. I was able to buy one, which had been advertised on our notice board for £15 by a lady specialist physician who worked in nearby Devonshire place. It is a beautiful monocular instrument: Leitz, Wetzlar 1898, which has accompanied me on all my travels. In September 1953 I began a year's appointment as senior house officer in the pathology laboratory of the Nottingham General Hospital and used microscopes daily in the haematology and bacteriology departments. In December 1954 I joined a private laboratory in Bulawayo, Southern Rhodesia, as an assistant to the pathologist, and again the microscope was an essential part of my daily work. When I opened my own general practice in Salisbury in 1970, I bought a binocular Olympus microscope. I was not certain about the services offered by the private laboratories and wanted to diagnose my own cases of malaria if they occurred in the middle of the night. I bought all the necessary equipment: a pestle and mortar, haematoxylin and eosin powder and methyl alcohol, and made my own stain. Several times, though during the daytime, I was able to see the parasites of malignant tertian malaria which still commonly occurred in that part of Africa at that time. Perhaps the most useful thing I learned from the senior technician at Nottingham was how to examine urines properly. Not only did this help me on numerous occasions to diagnose accurately cases of dysuria and lower abdominal pain, but I also found the parasites of urinary bilharzia, sexually transmitted trichomonas vaginalis and motile spermatozoa. This led me to do vaginal examinations and take fresh smears in normal saline, and I was able to calculate that motile sperms could live in the female genital tract for up to three days, while on two occasions I saw sickling in the red cells which had remained after a period. Skin diseases were common in the Europeans due to the sun. I missed the daily major surgery I had done in the government service and began to do minor surgery on the various skin lesions I met, which included taking biopsies and sending them to a laboratory. I bought all the equipment I would need, including a small autoclave to sterilise them. A friendly laboratory would send me a slide of the stained tissue with the diagnosis of each, and I was able to study the pathology of the lesions with my microscope and learn how to make the clinical diagnosis more accurately.

In England I began to examine the skeleton in 2017 and had made considerable progress but had to discontinue and do more work on my other book: The Foetal Circulation. I resumed work on the skeleton in early 2020. What interested me particularly was the pale, almost white material which covered parts of both surfaces of the vertebrae. I had paid little attention to this material and had only roughly sketched its outlines, but then I realised it deserved further study; I had never heard of

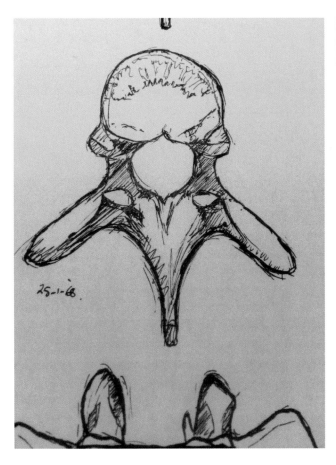 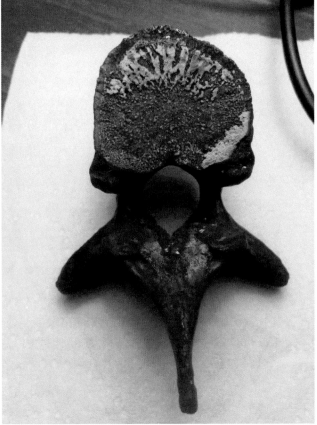

it before; what was it? See my drawing of the 8th dorsal vertebra from below, made in 1968, and my picture of the same bone taken recently.

I fetched my Olympus microscope and scanned the lower surface of the 4th dorsal vertebra with both 40 and 100 magnifications. I was surprised by what I saw. At 40 magnifications, using the 10 eyepiece and the 4 objective it was composed of irregular whitish masses of tiny pieces, which in places looked like rings, mainly round the perimeter of the surface. At 100 magnifications, using the 10 objective I confirmed that the pieces were rings, with a silvery covering which produced the whitish appearance at lower magnifications. In places, without the silvery covering, the rings were hyaline-looking, irregular with central holes, like little doughnuts, connected irregularly. Many of the rings were broken and parts of the rings were lying loose. The whole picture was of irregular whitish masses of little rings.

I put my plastic ruler, marked in millimetres, on the microscope stage and at 100 magnifications found that the diameter of my field of vision was 1.7mm, or 1700 microns. I then estimated (rather roughly you may guess), that about 50 rings would reach across the1700 microns of my visual field, that 100 rings would equal 3400 microns and that one ring would have a diameter of 34 microns. The diameter of the ring hole was about half that of the ring; say 17 microns, leaving plenty of room for red blood corpuscles with a diameter of 7.5 microns to pass through, with nerves and other things too.

I was very fortunate in having been able to contact James Charles; Director of Olympus, Glasgow, and was able buy from him another binocular microscope with improved features compared with those of my older one. This new one had a graticule and more lenses, and a camera which fitted into the right tube of my microscope. I took pictures with the camera and confirmed the appearances of the whitish masses and the rings which I had noted with my old microscope. See my pictures. The first shows the white masses at low magnification, while with the other at higher power, the rings

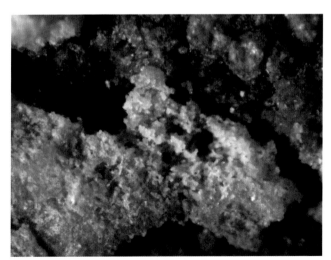 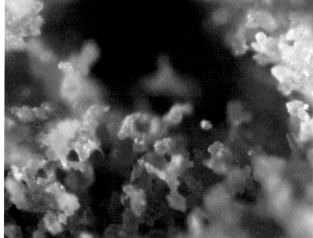

are clearly and beautifully shown.

At times 200 magnifications I was able to calculate that the diameter of the rings was nearer 60 microns, and that the diameter of the holes was a little more than a third of the diameter of the rings; say 25 microns. At first, I could not see the graticule clearly and it took some time before I could be sure of the measurements I had made. On rechecking the size of the rings in the 7th dorsal vertebra, I found the diameter of the rings to be 50 microns and the holes to be 20 microns in diameter. But the rings are irregular, and it depends on the shape of the rings; many are broken and only parts of the rings can be seen. I realised that there was a wide range of their sizes: some larger than those I had seen before, and many were much smaller. But they were all rings; there was no doubt about that. At the magnification of 100 I could see that the silvery covering was crystalline.

All the observations I had made were of the upper and lower surfaces of the vertebrae. I examined them further. The more superficial silvery white material was connected underneath to an amorphous brown layer, with an occasional crystal visible. In the more lateral part of this layer there were many small roundish elevations close together in irregular rows, while the more central area was smoother, and through gaps in each part of the surface could be seen a brown latticework structure with smooth edges which was the architecture of the central part of the vertebral body. By focusing up and down I was able to see that each of the three parts or layers of the surface, the pale material, the brown amorphous layer and the brown latticework, were all connected, each one to the next.

I wanted to see these three layers, not from above, but from the side, to see the relationship between them. I also wanted to see the architecture of the internal latticework. I had a small hacksaw with a blade which was only 0.5mm thick, and I sawed the 10th dorsal vertebra in half, from above down wards. I had missed the first layer of white crystals and only cut through the next two, and it was difficult to separate these two from the limiting wall of the latticework. With the graticule I measured the thickness of these two together to be between 100 and 125 microns. The sawing had revealed the internal architecture of the vertebra beautifully. See my picture. The bone here was brown in colour without any sparkling crystals. It was a latticework of arches with smooth edges and with oval or other shaped

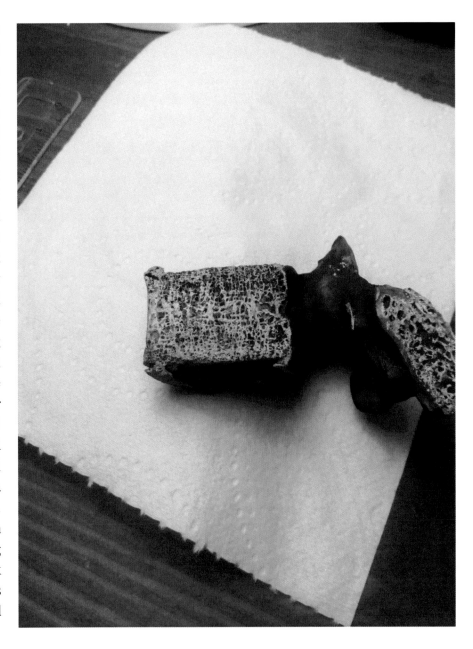

spaces between them. Where the spaces were tubular in shape the long axis of each tube was vertical, showing how the architecture of the body of the vertebra was able to resist the strength of the force applied to it above and below; rather like the columns in a cathedral which support the weight of the roof above. The varied pattern of the latticework would also be able to resist pressure from other directions. The cut ends of the latticework struts that I had sawn through had a rough silvery appearance. I examined the bony sawdust I had made. There were four features: large irregular conglomerates of whitish material, brown streaky material marked with the lines from the sawing, a background of small hyaline crystalline pieces and in some places a few tiny fibres. The first would have been bone crystals fused together, the brown streaky material would have been the outer covering of the bony latticework, while the small crystalline pieces would have broken off the large conglomerates. Here was revealed the nature of the bone in the interior of the vertebrae: a latticework of whitish crystals with a brown covering, which perhaps could be called cancellous. On using the graticule, I found one of the spaces to be 575 microns in diameter, and some of the oval tubular spaces were even longer. The latticework reached right up close to the layer of bone above and fused with it, as I have shown earlier. In fact, the upper limiting layer of the latticework was also the upper surface of the vertebra, just as the lower end of the latticework was also the lower surface of the vertebra. In the centre of the posterior wall of this vertebra was a large funnel shaped hole, 7 mm. across at the surface with the openings of the lattice work leading into it, which undoubtedly would have led into the basi-vertebral vein. Scattered round the outside wall were several small holes, mostly nearer the upper surface, which would have been the entrances of the periosteal arteries, some supplying the bony outer wall and some supplying the internal architecture. See my picture. It is quite easy to see the latticework through the larger holes with the naked eye, some of the larger holes measuring more than

1 mm. in diameter. In the darkened and dim light of my bedroom at night I pointed a penlight torch into the holes and was able to see some light in the posterior funnel. I also shone the light from the cut surface of the latticework and could see light in the periosteal holes. I filled a 5 ml. syringe with water, and using the attached needle injected some into the larger holes. Each time it quickly came dropping out through the posterior funnel, and though it would not pass through the upper and lower surfaces of the vertebra, I expect the oxygen supply for each surface would have been adequate. The spaces within the latticework would have been filled in life with red marrow, supplied with blood from the arteries of the periosteum. The interior of the vertebrae, therefore, consists of two quite different materials: the bony framework and the red marrow, with two quite different functions: physical support and haemopoiesis, both supplied by the periosteal arteries, and both draining venous blood posteriorly into

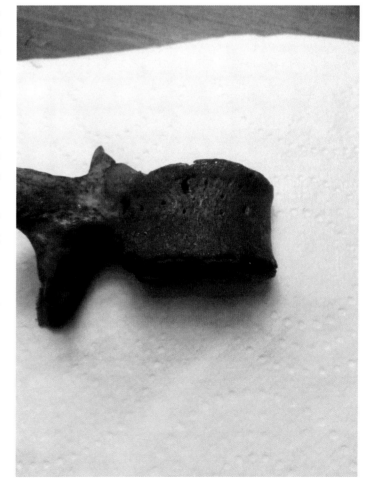

the basi-vertebral vein. It is important to realise that the framework of the latticework is not sealed in within the bone. It would prevent a circulation within the vertebral body. All the spaces are interconnected and connect with the holes in the wall and the funnel-shaped opening at the rear. In life, there would have been a circulation of blood, nourishing the bone and haemopoetic tissue, beginning with arterial blood in the periosteal arteries and ending with venous blood flowing into the funnel shaped opening and the basi-vertebral vein.

At 40 times magnification I scanned the whole of the outside wall of the half vertebra and followed it up to each end without finding any evidence of rings. The walls of the vertebrae are not straight vertical; they are curved concave so that at each end there is an acute angle of bone which has two components: below is the end of the outer wall and perched on top of it is a plate of smooth material which may also be bone. In places the two are fused together, but elsewhere there are gaps between the two. This arrangement runs right round the top of the rim of the vertebra and is *the annular epiphysis* we are meeting for the first time. The gaps would probably have been filled in life with hyaline cartilage. We have caught a stage in the formation of the vertebral epiphysis which had almost been completed, showing us that this mature teen age girl had almost stopped growing and almost become a young lady.

In two places I was able to pass a 5 amp. fuse wire (.2 mm thick), in the gap between the outer wall and the plate above it, but in most of the gaps the wire would only enter a short distance and be blocked. In those places where the upper plate had broken off, I could see that the broken pieces would have extended a few mm. towards the centre of the vertebral surface. There were two layers of the whitish material associated with the epiphysis: a lower one which extended from the inner border of the outer wall and lay on the surface of the bone, and the upper one which extended inwardly from the upper plate of the epiphysis, to meet the lower. The two outlined the wedged-shape cross section of the epiphysis, with the base on the outer wall and the apex pointing to the centre of the surface. See my diagram.

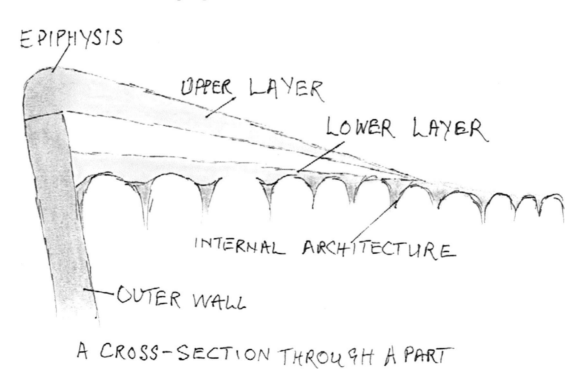

A CROSS-SECTION THROUGH A PART
OF THE END OF THE VERTEBRA

I had already begun, early in the year, to work out a plan of the growth and development of the vertebrae, but an important thing I had learned during the years I had spent working on my other book, was the world of difference between an observation and an opinion of it. One is valuable, the other questionable: the difference between fact and fiction. On making an observation it is important to observe carefully and critically, and to record one's findings accurately shortly afterwards on the same day; anything added later loses value. (I sometimes forget to do this). Then any theory or hypothesis concerning the observation must be supported with evidence such as by experiment, or from the work of others. Let me show you, my ideas.

There is a fourth layer missing in the vertebrae of the girl who had died: most probably hyaline cartilage, which I will now call the first layer. I have assumed it would have lain across each end of the bone during her lifetime, and laid down the hyaline cartilage rings, which would quickly absorb crystals of the bone salts and form the second, crystalline whitish layer. This would then be changed into the brown amorphous third layer, which would develop into the latticework in the centre of the vertebral body. In this manner, both ends of the vertebra would grow in the same way that modern high-rise buildings grow, with new materials being added from above (and below).

For support, I needed to examine living, growing vertebrae and see if there were the four layers. On the human and even on living animals it was out of the question, but with meat from the butcher which had been preserved by freezing it seemed feasible. Kevin Battams, of Battams Butchery Oswestry, kindly gave me the lumbar vertebrae of a three-month old lamb. It takes a year for lambs to become sheep, and without doubt this lamb had been growing. I removed the last two vertebrae by cutting through the intervertebral disc above them and placed them in diluted formalin. I then removed half of the next vertebra above by sawing across the middle of the bone and replaced the remainder in the freezer. The next day I sawed vertically downwards through the half vertebra, cutting off a quarter of the bone and was able to view the layers of the lower surface from the side. I could not see any rings. I was very disappointed, but it meant that there were other things to find, which I had not even dreamed about. Running across the bone, just over 1 mm. from the surface was a wavy bluish line which had a shiny, jelly-like or watery appearance. It separated what appeared to be the epiphysis, from the shaft of the bone. I put this quarter of the vertebra back in the freezer and left the other quarter on my desk for the night. The next day the freezer specimen still carried the blue line, though it was not so shiny, but the line had disappeared from the other bone left out overnight, leaving a thin dark gap between the shaft and the epiphysis. What did this mean? I do not think the thin blue line would have been cartilage; three months in the ground to disappear I can accept, but not 15 hours in the air. However, perhaps the growth of the vertebrae in a lamb is fundamentally the same as in the human, but the materials used are different. In which case in both, a layer of special material, either cartilage or something different, would lay down the latticework of the bony shaft below, with the epiphysis above. Like the growth of the high-rise buildings, as I have said. But why the epiphysis; high-rise buildings do not have epiphyses? *Because the lamb and the human have begun to have the function of the mature bone prematurely, while they are still growing.* (Unlike the high-rise buildings which do not add the special features at the top until they have finished growing).

I removed the rest of the vertebral column from the freezer and sawed across the middle of the next full vertebra above, capturing the intervertebral disc lying between one half vertebra above and another half vertebra below. I then sawed down through the middle of the specimen in an antero-posterior plane and exposed the disc and the two adjacent epiphyses.

I sawed off the end of part of the vertebra which had been preserved in formalin, then sawed vertically across the disc. The blue material between the epiphysis and the shaft had been preserved, and anteriorly was thick. I shaved some of it off, viewed it under the microscope and took two pictures. It resembled the skin of a strawberry, with little pits in the surface. Between the pits I could imagine them connected by rings of the blue material, 50 microns in diameter! Were these the equivalent of the rings in the vertebrae of my Zimbabwe skeleton? See my picture.

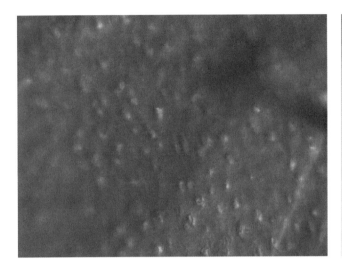 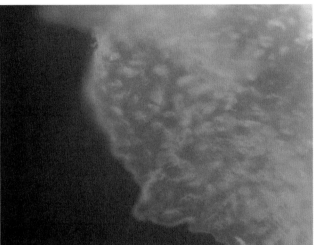

I left the specimen out overnight and it dried up somewhat. In the morning I scraped more off and viewed the pieces at times 40 and 100. The pits were now little blobs without surrounding connecting material but were about 50 microns apart. I took another picture.

This was great news! There was similarity between the lamb and human vertebrae. The little pits or blobs were of the same size as the rings in the young lady's vertebrae and came from the same region above the bone shaft below. Were the rings and blobs, therefore, not made by the cartilage and changed into bone with the aquisition of bone salts?

I re-examined the surfaces of the Zim vertebrae: the pale material, which I call immature bone, was limited to the periphery, near the epiphysyses; the more central parts were clear of the pale bone and smoother. I put the eleventh dorsal vertebra on the stage and examined the central upper surface. At times 40, many small holes and gaps of various sizes appeared across the rough brownish surface. At times 100 superficially, it was an amber irregular latticework covered in silvery crystals. Focussing deeper there was an abundance of small roundish hyaline or whitish blobs or crystals, which covered the brownish latticework of the central architechture. I took pictures of both levels at times 100.

During the night, a small spider had laid a web across the objectives of my microscope. I examined one thread at times 100. It was 30 microns wide. I took a picture.

I examined the central areas of both surfaces of the 3rd to 7th cervical vertebrae, at times 40 and 100. The lower magnification was useful to identify the central areas correctly, while the higher revealed the features at each level. At times 40 there were a few thin curved fibres, 20 microns in diameter and thinner than the spider's web, while at times 100 there were numerous tiny straight fibres running in all directions, with some of them no thicker than the finest markings of the graticule. The findings were similar throughout the five bones, with the surface having three regions from superficial to deep connected gradually without a barrier between them. The most superficial structure was irregular, covered in small silvery crystals, with scattered holes through which I could see the deeper parts. There was a gradual transition as I focussed lower, with fewer crystals and more regular features, leading to the brownish latticework which still contained some crystals superficially. The fine adjustment of the microscope was marked in divisions from 0 to 200. I supposed they represented microns; in which case this surface region was about 200 microns deep.

I had thought that there would be four layers at each end of a growing vertebra with the second pale bone changing into the more mature bone below. But the pale bone appears to be part of the epiphysis only and not a precusor of the more central region of the surface. In which case the second layer would be absent in the centre and the cartilage plate would lay down the third layer directly without the intervention of the second pale layer containing the rings. Why therefore is it necessary to form the epiphysis from the hyaline rings? That is the essential problem which confronts me!

The vertebral column had come from a large girl who was still growing, and her vertebrae were performing the functions of the mature skeleton prematurely. Let us look at the intervertebral discs.

Between cartilages of two adjacent vertebrae there is a special connective tissue feature which both separates and joins the two together. Peripherally, strong collagenous fibres join the outer rim of each bone to the other. This is the annulus fibrosus. Within this fibrous rim or ring, is the nucleus pulposus. It contains a fluid-like jelly which separates the two vertebrae and carries the weight of the one on the other. The weight is transferred in the fluid laterally to the annulus fibrosus which pulls the vertebrae together; the epiphyses do not bear weight. *The nucleus keeps the bones apart and allows movement between them; the annulus keeps them together and restricts movement.* With the lower magnification, in places round the perimeter of the vertebrae can be seen the grooves made by the strong anchoring fibres of the annulus. Also, round the perimeter the pale bone and rings have a streaky pattern, probably caused by other fibres, pointing towards the centre, and at the edges the streakiness is more angled in line with the edge of the bone.

I have made several observations; what do they all mean? It is complicated. The pale immature bone, made up of masses of rings, is without doubt associated with the epiphyses, all of which lie on the periphery. Do the rings change into the more mature bone of the epiphyses, and do the rings make the anchoring fibres? The strong anchoring fibres have disappeared, probably because they were collagenous. But the tiny fibres have not disappeared; are they inorganic?

In life, the layer of hyaline cartilage would have spread right across the surface of the vertebra, not only above the thick layer of pale bone, but below it too until it had reached the outer wall, separating from the rest of the vertebra a ring of pale bone, *which is the epiphysis.* The cartilage plate would therefore have split into two layers: one above the epiphysis and one below. When the skeleton had finished growing, the lower layer would have disappeared, and the epiphysis would have completely joined the main part of the vertebra. X-rays of a mature vertebral column show how the epiphyses have disappeared

Today, 9th of July, I have begun to try to describe the vertebrae better, beginning with the 3rd to 7th cervical. The upper and lower surfaces are similar. I divide each into three regions: the outer rim of the mature bone of the epiphysis, inside which is the pale immature bone, and the central area of mature bone. These can be seen clearly with the naked eye, and the rim looks smooth. But at times 40 the rim has a more granular appearance and some of the 'granules' are ring-shaped. At the higher magnification of 100 there is a deeper smooth amber layer overlaid with rougher irregular particles and rings glistening in the reflected light of my bright spotlight. On the inner side of the rim are a few gaps through which can be seen parts of the bony latticework. The latticework comes right up to the rim, underneath the pale bone. In some places the outermost part of the rim is darker in colour, almost purplish. I examined both surfaces of all the dorsal vertebrae, including the tenth which I had sawed in half, in the same manner, with findings similar to those of the cervical bones.

On the upper surface of lumbar 2 anteriorly the rim is covered with two layers of pale bone. The deeper layer on the surface has many rings loosely connected. The superficial layer is different; the rings are fewer and distorted in a more- streaky sort of pattern. This indicates to me that the upper layer is more mature than the lower. Viewed from the outside, the two layers of the mature bone have not quite fused together. Where they have fused the pale bone seems to have become one layer. I must check this out very carefully tomorrow.

It is tricky; very difficult to work out what happens in life. The pale bone spreads a long way round the inner part of the rim and projections lead from it towards the centre of the surface, getting smaller and thinner and ending short of the central region. There are grooves in the surface of some of the bones and the pale bone projections occupy them.

Today, 11th July, I investigated the pale bone of the upper surface of D 8. Where there were rings clearly seen, I considered the bone to be recently formed. Where the rings were less obvious and included in a streaky sort of material, I thought the bone would have been laid down earlier. I scanned the streaks of pale bone running to the centre of the surface; the rings were clearer near the periphery and less clear near the centre. If the rings had been laid down by cartilage the process would have started centrally without rings and spread outwards, laying down more rings in the process. Was the pale bone continuous with the underlying bone or separated from it? With my penknife I chipped a piece of the pale bone off from the more peripheral part and examined it under the microscope. On the upper surface there were many rings; underneath there was part of the latticework I had chipped off. *The pale immature bone was continuous with the latticework below and there was no evidence of cartilage between the two.* I took pictures and kept the specimen.

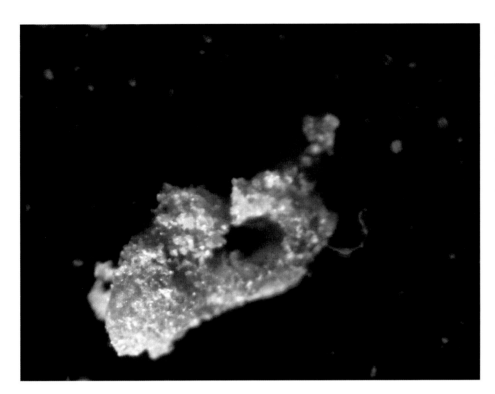

These two pictures, at low and high power, show the pale bone on the upper part of the chip.

The next two pictures, also at low and high power, show a part of the internal latticework of the vertebra.

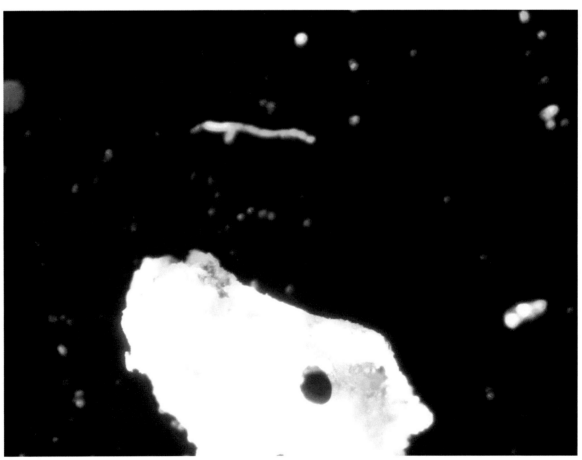

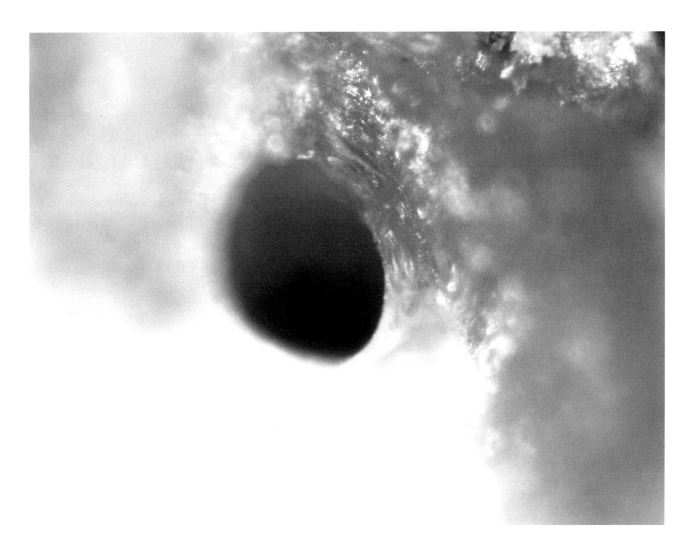

These pictures, of upper and lower views of the tiny chip at low and higher magnifications, show that the pale bone and the latticework are fused together. The upper surface of the vertebra without the pale bone, and the upper limiting wall of the latticework, are one and the same thing.

So how did the cartilage create the vertebra?

It seems to me that the cartilage would have started in the centre, laying down a thin layer of hyaline rings which rapidly absorbed salts and changed into the latticework. The process would spread out all round and in parts begun to make a thicker column of rings. When the columns were near the periphery the cartilage would have divided into two layers, laying down rings all the time. The top layer would form the upper part of the outer wall, while the lower layer would reach the outer wall below the other, creating the epiphysis between them. At maturity the lower cartilage layer would have changed into bone and the epiphysis joined the main bone.

I will now try to summarise the structure of the human vertebral body brought over from Zimbabwe.

It is a column of bone, somewhat D or kidney shaped in cross section, joined to the pedicles at each corner posteriorly, with each end having the same structural pattern. The interior is formed of a framework or latticework of bony strands, vertical and lateral, crossing each other with spaces in between. It reaches to the outer wall and both end surfaces, inseparably joined to them all. The thin outer wall is vertically concave, ending above and below in an acute angle. There are many small holes in the wall, mainly in the upper part, which connect with the interior spaces. The spaces are not sealed off but connect freely with the larger spaces of the central region leading to a funnel-shaped gap in the posterior wall, which is the beginning of the basi-vertebral vein. Here is revealed the path taken by the blood supply for the interior of the vertebra: from the periosteal arteries to the latticework and the basi-vertebral vein, more effective when the spine is in the erect position. Running round each end of the outer wall, above and below, is a ring of bone which is the epiphysis. In places it joins the wall but elsewhere there are gaps between them. In some places the epiphysis has broken off, revealing streaks of pale bone on the surface leading towards the surface centre. Where the epiphysis is intact it connects with more pale bone leading to the centre above the other and joining the other at its termination. The central part of the surface is relatively smooth, but the region nearer the outer wall contains many small bumps caused by the underlying internal framework. Some of the bumps have the tops broken off, revealing the uppermost part of the internal architecture which is easily seen with the microscope. I have assumed that in life a plate of hyaline cartilage would have spread across the surface and split into two layers to cover the upper and lower surfaces of the epiphysis.(If the plate of cartilage is able to produce the smoother bone in the centre without pale bone as an intermediary, why is it necessary to make the epiphysis with the pale bone; why is it necessary to create an epiphysis? I still do not know the answer). Between cartilages of two adjacent vertebrae there is a special connective tissue feature which both separates and joins the two together. Peripherally, strong fibres join the outer rim of each bone to the other. This is the annulus fibrosus. Within this fibrous rim or ring, is the nucleus pulposus. It contains a fluid-like jelly which separates the two vertebrae and carries the weight of the one on the other. Under the low power only a few small fibres can be seen, but round the periphery there are several grooves and imprints left by the strong fibres of the annulus fibrosus, while with the higher power there are many tiny, short fibres scattered throughout.

The internal architecture of the vertebra gives it strength with little weight. Even when full of blood with a specific gravity close to that of water (1.06), it is still a lightweight structure. Attached posteriorly to the upper part of each corner of the 'D' are two strong pedicles which lead on each side to superior and inferior articular facets, laminae and transverse processes. The two laminae, completing with the pedicles and vertebral body the spinal canal for the spinal cord and nerves, fuse together to form the posterior spinal process. The spinal and transverse processes are strong levers, which in the living have muscles attached which move the spine, while the smooth cartilage- covered articular processes smoothly glide together and guide and limit the movements. Between adjacent vertebrae there is a foramen on each side under the pedicles which transmit the spinal nerves. Each dorsal vertebra has a costal element on each side, which are the ribs attached to the bodies of adjacent vertebrae and the transverse processes, and which curve round anteriorly to form the skeleton of the thorax. In the cervical vertebrae the costal element is the anterior part of the foramen transversarium, while in the lumbar vertebrae it is the transverse process. I sawed off an articular process from D 10 vertebra and viewed the surface with times 100 of the microscope. Though smooth to the naked eye, under the microscope it was irregular with ridges and furrows, which I suppose would have helped to secure the overlain cartilage. The ridges were bluish with small particles which shone in the light of my spotlight, like crystals. In the depth of the furrows the colour was the normal of brown bone, while the small particles did not shine in the shadows.

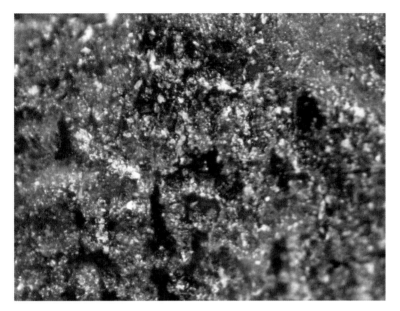

These small particles, embedded in the bony matrix, measured from 20 microns across to 5 microns or even less. I sawed across the articular surface and examined the internal structure: it was similar to the internal architecture of the vertebral body. There are three pictures here of the articular surface. The first gives a low power view showing the ridges and furrows, the second is high power superficial and the third is high power deeper.

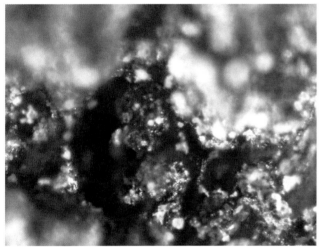

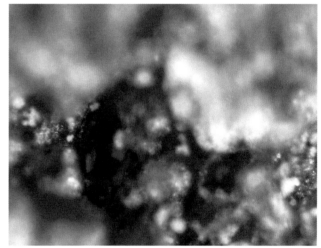

On 14-7-2020, I sawed through the small part of D 10, and was able to cut through all three layers, as well as cutting through the thicker layer too. All three layers were fused to the latticework, and the top thicker layer was fused to the lower three and the latticework. During the sawing, a piece of the top layer broke off. I put it on the slide next to the main bone where it had broken off. Later, I took pictures of it with the camera. Below are the pictures at low and high magnification. (Times 40 and 100). With the graticule, I estimated the diameter of the rings to be 60-70 microns, and the holes to be 20-30 microns across. So what would have filled the spaces between the rings, tissue fluid?

15-7. It is not easy to understand the vertebral surfaces; it is very difficult. It has to be taken one step at a time. I call the epiphysis the outermost ring of smooth mature bone which runs right round on top of the outer wall. Without doubt, the pale bone is associated with the epiphysis. There are two layers, upper and lower. The lower extends in streaks from the inside of the outer wall halfway towards the centre and is fused with the underlying bone. The upper is fused to the epiphysis and extends centrally sloping down to fuse with the lower. I think it fair to include each part of the pale

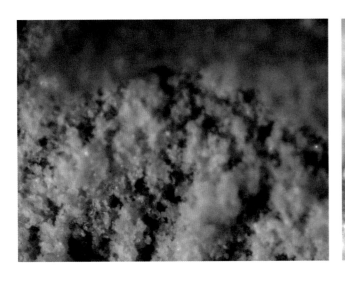
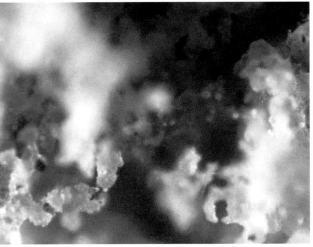

bone with the epiphysis. See this diagram and the pictures of the upper and lower surfaces of the 9th dorsal vertebra.

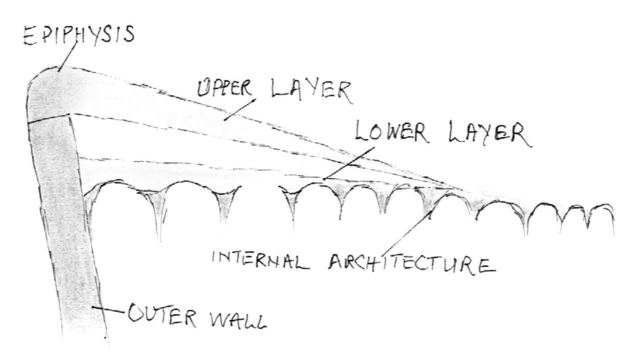

EPIPHYSIS

UPPER LAYER

LOWER LAYER

INTERNAL ARCHITECTURE

OUTER WALL

A CROSS-SECTION THROUGH A PART OF THE END OF THE VERTEBRA

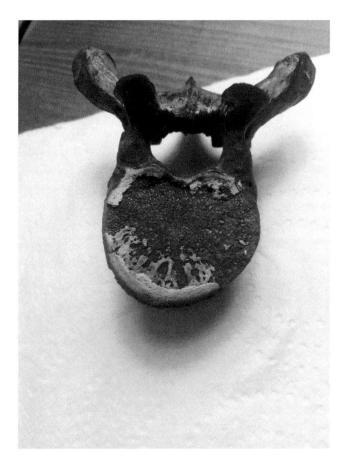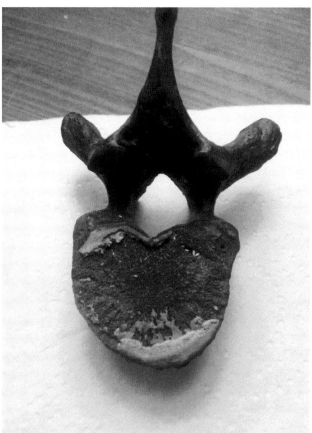

There are many features of the skeleton I had brought over from Africa which require investigation. At present I am trying to understand why we have epiphyses, but some of the other features must be included in my story because they might have a bearing on this topic. Many of the forensic cases which I had been involved with in Fort Victoria in the 1960's, resulted in my giving evidence in the magistrates' court. The more serious cases, such as this one, were later heard in the high court, which came down to Fort Victoria six times a year. I was not then able to give the cause of death, but now, many years later and with more time to study the skeleton at leisure, I believe the girl had been burnt to death. There is clear evidence of burning on several of the bones. I did not follow up this case and do not know what the outcome was. But it seems probable to me that she may not have had a just and honourable conclusion for herself and her family. If there had been a fire, why was her death reported to the police three months later? It is unlikely that the fire would not have been seen by the villagers. I am sorry if I have let her down by not giving the correct cause of death.

The burning may have altered some of the tissues which had survived; some may have been preserved better, others less well. On the 3rd 4th and 5th lumbar vertebrae, much of the annulus fibrosus has been preserved in a dried mummified-like state. It is like a very dark blue membrane. See my pictures of the upper and lower surfaces of the 3rd lumbar vertebra. Below them is a side view of the 4th and 5th lumbar vertebrae joined, and the lower surface of the 5th lumbar.

I snipped a small piece off the annulus fibrosus from the 3rd lumbar vertebra and examined it under the low and high power of the microscope. At times 100 the thickest fibres measured a little more than one division, say 15 microns. I had assumed that the parallel markings on the epiphysis were grooves formerly occupied by the fibres of the annulus fibrosus. I examined the epiphysis on the lower surface of the 9th dorsal vertebra and measured the grooves there.

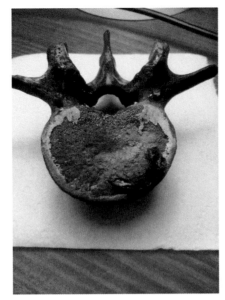
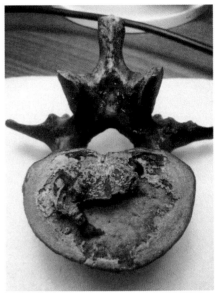

They were a little more than two divisions in diameter, say 25 microns.

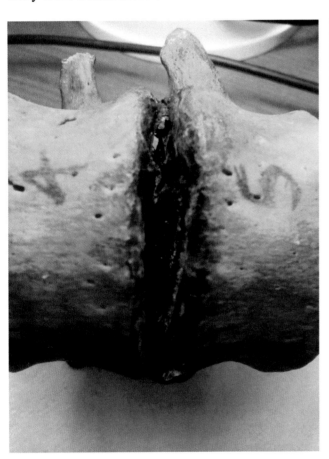
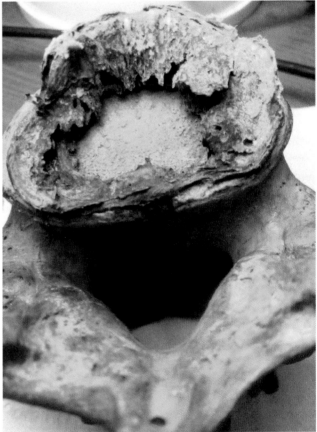

It is important to investigate the annulus fibrosus; it is intimately related to the epiphysis. I have studied both surfaces of all the vertebrae, except the first two which are atypical, the 10th dorsal which I had sawn in half and the 4th and 5th lumbar joined by the annulus. With the microscope at times 40 magnifications, I examined every part of every piece of the mature bone of the epiphysis. On each one there were either grooves, fibres or parallel markings which could only have been made by fibres. *The fibres of the annulus*

fibrosus were invariably attached to the epiphysis. But some extended inwardly to the upper layer of pale bone. Some were on the lower pale bone layer, or even on the surface below it, and a few were found on the outer wall of the vertebrae. It would seem that the function of the epiphysis is to provide a strong imbedding for the annulus to keep the bones together.

One does not need a microscope to see the extensive origin of the annulus from the outer wall, the mature epiphysis and the lower surface of the 5th lumbar vertebra. Here we have been fortunate to capture the two layers of the annulus which would have enclosed the nucleus pulposus of the strong lumbo-sacral joint.

Though single grooves or fibres may be found, they are mostly in rows, each lying parallel side by side with the next. They lie in various directions, mostly at right angles to the line of the epiphysis and pointing to the centre of the vertebral surface. But some are in line with the epiphysis and others lie obliquely at various angles to it. On the right posterior corner of the lower surface of the 4th cervical vertebra there is a mass of grooves or fibres lying in all directions. In my experience, the cervical disc which suffers most in various clinical situations is the one between the 5th and 6th cervical vertebrae. In this case it would have been the next disc above.

Most African village ladies carry buckets of water and other heavy loads on their heads; it is their normal lifestyle. Here we see the evidence of it.

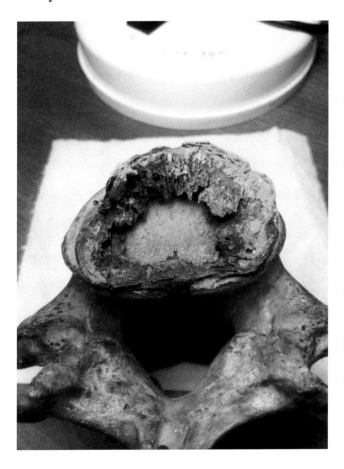 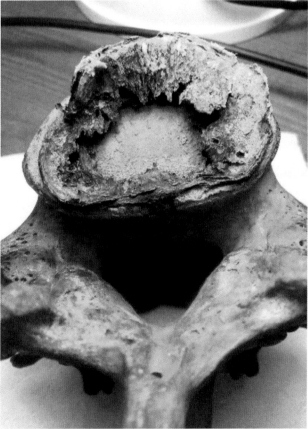

30 May 2024. Two interesting things happened when I was in Fort Victoria. I had found the most important evidence on the foetal circulation, which contradicted all the orthodox accounts, and I was allowed to keep the skeleton of a teen-age girl which carried many epiphyses. When I returned to England in 2013,

after having spent 59 years in Africa, I had the desire to investigate four things: the foetal circulation, the epiphysis, balance, and vision.

I began with the epiphysis, and you can see from the several pages above, that I had made good progress. But I was living in Oswestry near the border with Wales and I was able to find a sheep farmer who gave me several stillborn lambs which helped me to understand the foetal circulation. I therefore stopped my work on the epiphysis and devoted all my spare time to the investigation of the foetal circulation.

At that time, I was living with my son Andrew and his wife Kim and their sons, and there was little room for me to dissect my specimens. After some years, I was able to move into a flat with more room. I bought a freezer and kept my specimens in it. I managed to publish four editions of my book on the foetal circulation, while I was in Oswestry, but they gave me no financial return. Not only was my bank balance in a poor state, but my physical balance was not very good either. In June 2022, I had a stroke and spent a month in hospital. On returning to my flat, Andrew thought I should not be living by myself, and my daughter Mary and her husband Bernard Kirkman, invited me to live with them in Horley Surrey. On 24th September that year, Andrew drove me down to Horley, and I began to receive the most generous and loving care imaginable. I had already begun to write a much better 8th edition of my book and by April 2024, I was waiting to receive the first copy from the publisher.

I began to enjoy the new-found freedom without anything to write, and Bernard and Mary, with three children, three dogs, and two cats, and me, were all whisked away to Northampton on 17th May this year. We landed in a beautiful home in 2 Meadow Sweet Road Rushden. I have woken up from my happiness today and have even begun to think more about the epiphysis.

Today, 7th June, 2024, I have begun to investigate the epiphysis. I had separated the bones of the left side of the African skeleton from the rest, and I would only dissect the bones of the left side. I am trying to find if the rings occur in the other epiphysies, in those not connected to the vertebrae, and which part of the skeleton can really be called an epiphysis?

Today, 1st of September 2024, I am still waiting for the 8th edition of my first book to be published, and complications have arrived. For several months I have had an anaemia. A CT scan show a cancer in my ascending colon. I want it removed as soon as possible, but I am told by the surgical specialist that I may not be fit for the anaesthetic. I am in crisis. I may have only a few weeks to live. The 8th edition will be published, whether or not I will be alive to see it, but I have to make sure that my small second book will be published too, even though I might not be alive. There is much of scientific interest in the book to make it publishable, but I will try to add more while I am able.

Alan.

Printed in the United States
by Baker & Taylor Publisher Services